Green Keto Recipes

A Collection Super Healthy Vegetable-Based Keto Recipes

By Carla Wilson

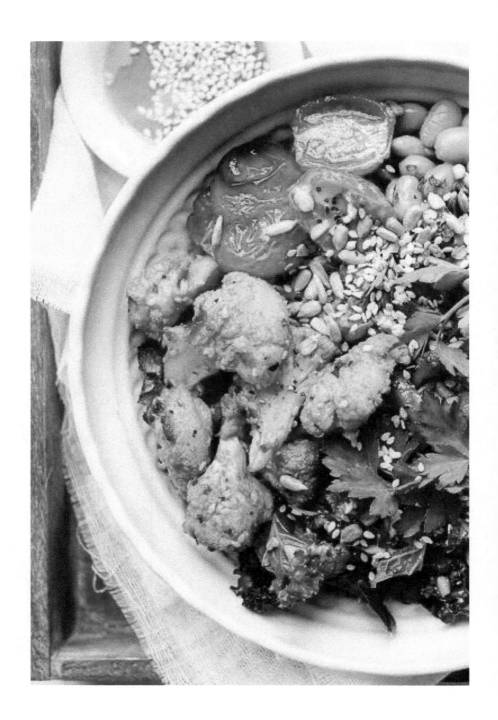

content within this book has been derived from various sources. Please consult a licensed professional before attempting any techniques outlined in this book.

By reading this document, the reader agrees that under no circumstances is the author responsible for any losses, direct or indirect, which are incurred as a result of the use of information contained within this document, including, but not limited to, — errors, omissions, or inaccuracies.

Table of Contents

Italian Stuffed Mushrooms

Preparation Time: 10 minutes

Cooking Time: 35 minutes

Servings: 4

Ingredients:

- 1-pound button mushrooms, stems removed
- 2 tablespoons coconut oil, melted
- 1-pound broccoli florets
- 1 Italian pepper, chopped
- 1 teaspoon Italian herb mix
- Salt and pepper, to taste
- 1 shallot, finely chopped
- 2 garlic cloves, minced
- 1 cup vegan parmesan

Directions:

1. Parboil the broccoli in a large pot of salted water until crisp-tender, about 6 minutes. Mash the broccoli florets with a potato masher. In a saucepan, melt the coconut oil over a moderately-high heat. Once hot, cook the shallot, garlic, and pepper until tender and fragrant. Season with the spices and add in the broccoli.

2. Fill the mushroom cups with the broccoli mixture and bake in the preheated oven at 365 degrees F for about 10 minutes. Top with the vegan parmesan and bake for 10 minutes more or until it melts.

Nutrition:

- 206 Calories
- 13.4g Fat
- 12.7g Protein
- 4g Fiber

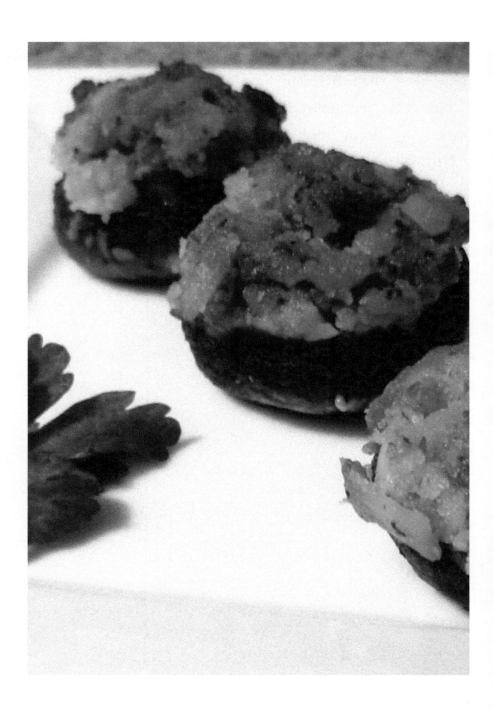

One-Pot Mushroom Stroganoff

Preparation Time: 10 minutes

Cooking Time: 25 minutes

Serving: 4

Ingredients:

- 2 tablespoons canola oil
- 1 parsnip, chopped
- 1 cup fresh brown mushrooms, sliced
- 1 cup onions, chopped
- 2 garlic cloves, pressed
- 1/2 cup celery rib, chopped
- 1 teaspoon Hungarian paprika
- 3 ½ cups roasted vegetable broth
- 1 cup tomato puree
- 1 tablespoon flaxseed meal
- 2 tablespoons sherry wine
- 1 rosemary sprig, chopped
- 1/2 teaspoon dried basil
- 1/2 teaspoon dried oregano

Directions:

1. In a heavy-bottomed pot, heat the oil over a moderately-high flame. Cook the onion and garlic for 2 minutes or until tender and aromatic.
2. Add in the celery, parsnip, and mushrooms, and continue to cook until they've softened; reserve.
3. Add in the sherry wine to deglaze the bottom of your pot. Add in the seasonings, vegetable broth, and tomato puree.
4. Continue to simmer, partially covered, for 15 to 18 minutes. Add in the flaxseed meal and stir until the sauce has thickened.

Nutrition:

- 114 Calories
- 7.3g Fat
- 2.1g Protein 3.1g Fiber

Avocado with Pine Nuts

Preparation Time: 5 minutes

Cooking Time: 10 minutes

Serving: 4

Ingredients:

- 2 avocados, pitted and halved
- 1 tablespoon coconut aminos
- 1/2 teaspoon garlic, minced
- 1 teaspoon fresh lime juice
- Salt and pepper, to taste
- 5 ounces pine nuts, ground
- 1 celery stalk, chopped

Directions:

1. Thoroughly combine the avocado pulp with the pine nuts, celery, garlic, fresh lime juice, and coconut aminos. Season with salt and pepper to taste.
2. Spoon the filling into the avocado halves.

Nutrition:

- 263 Calories
- 24.8g Fat
- 3.5g Protein
- 6.1g Fiber

Zucchini Noodles with Famous Cashew Parmesan

Preparation Time: 5 minutes

Cooking Time: 15 minutes

Serving: 4

Ingredients:

For Zoodles:

- 2 tablespoons canola oil
- 4 zucchinis, peeled and sliced into noodle-shape strands
- Salt and pepper, to taste

For Cashew Parmesan:

- 1/2 cup raw cashews
- 1/4 teaspoon onion powder
- 1 garlic clove, minced
- 2 tablespoons nutritional yeast
- Sea salt and pepper, to taste

Directions:

1. In a saucepan, heat the canola oil over medium heat; once hot, cook your zoodles for 1 minute or so, stirring frequently to ensure even cooking.
2. Season with salt and pepper to taste.

3. In your food processor, process all ingredients for the cashew parmesan. Toss the cashew parmesan with the zoodles and enjoy!

Nutrition:

- 145 Calories
- 10.6g Fat
- 5.5g Protein
- 1.6g Fiber

Cream of Broccoli Soup

Preparation Time: 5 minutes

Cooking Time: 15 minutes

Serving: 4

Ingredients:

- 1-pound broccoli, cut into small florets
- 8 ounces baby spinach
- 4 cups roasted vegetable broth
- 2 tablespoons olive oil
- 1 yellow onion, chopped
- 2 garlic cloves, minced
- 1/2 cup coconut milk
- Salt and pepper, to taste
- 2 tablespoons parsley, chopped

Directions:

1. Heat the oil in a soup pot over a moderately-high flame. Then, sauté the onion and garlic until they're tender and fragrant.
2. Add in the broccoli, spinach, and broth; bring to a rolling boil. Immediately turn the heat to a simmer.
3. Pour in the coconut milk, salt, pepper, and parsley; continue to simmer, partially covered, until cooked through.

18

4.   Puree your soup with an immersion blender.

Nutrition:

- 252 Calories20.3g Fat
- 8.1g Protein
- 4.5g Fiber

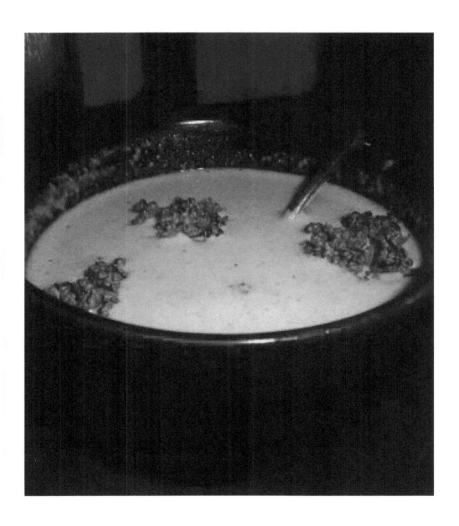

Swiss Chard Chips with Avocado Dip

Preparation Time: 10 minutes

Cooking Time: 20 minutes

Serving: 6

Ingredients:

- 1 tablespoon coconut oil
- Sea salt and pepper, to taste
- 2 cups Swiss chard, cleaned

Avocado Dip:

- 3 ripe avocados, pitted and mashed
- 2 garlic cloves, finely minced
- 2 tablespoons extra-virgin olive oil
- 2 teaspoons lemon juice
- Salt and pepper, to taste

Directions:

1. Toss the Swiss chard with the coconut oil, salt, and pepper. Bake the Swiss chard leaves in the preheated oven at 310 degrees F for about 10 minutes until the edges brown but are not burnt.
2. Thoroughly combine the ingredients for the avocado dip.

Nutrition:

- 269 Calories
- 26.7g Fat
- 2.3g Protein
- 4.1g Fiber

Banana Blueberry Smoothie

Preparation Time: 5 minutes

Cooking Time: 0 minutes

Serving: 4

Ingredients:

- 1/2 cup fresh blueberries
- 1/2 banana, peeled and sliced
- 1/2 cup water
- 1 ½ cups coconut milk
- 1 tablespoon vegan protein powder, zero carbs

Directions:

1. Blend all ingredients until creamy and uniform.

Nutrition:

- 247 Calories
- 21.7g Fat
- 2.6g Protein
- 3g Fiber

Cajun Artichoke with Tofu

Preparation Time: 15 minutes

Cooking Time: 30 minutes

Serving: 4

Ingredients:

- 1-pound artichokes, trimmed and cut into pieces
- 2 tablespoons coconut oil, room temperature
- 1 block tofu, pressed and cubed
- 1 teaspoon fresh garlic, minced
- 1 teaspoon Cajun spice mix
- 1 Spanish pepper, chopped
- 1/4 cup vegetable broth
- Salt and pepper, to taste

Directions:

1. Parboil your artichokes in a pot of lightly salted water for 13 to 15 minutes or until they're crisp-tender; drain.
2. In a large saucepan, melt the coconut oil over medium-high heat; fry the tofu cubes for 5 to 6 minutes or until golden-brown.
3. Add in the garlic, Cajun spice mix, Spanish pepper, broth, salt, and pepper. Add in the reserved artichokes and continue to cook until for 5 minutes more.

23

Nutrition:

- 138 Calories
- 8.9g Fat
- 6.4g Protein
- 5g Fiber

Mushroom and Cauliflower Medley

Preparation Time: 15 minutes

Cooking Time: 30 minutes

Serving: 4

Ingredients:

- 8 ounces brown mushrooms, halved
- 1 head cauliflower, cut into florets
- 1/4 cup olive oil
- 1/2 teaspoon turmeric powder
- 1 teaspoon garlic, smashed
- 1 cup tomato, pureed
- Salt and pepper, to taste

Directions:

1. Toss all ingredients in a lightly oiled baking pan.
2. Roast the vegetable in the preheated oven at 380 degrees F for 25 to 30 minutes.

Nutrition:

- 113 Calories
- 6.7g Fat
- 5g Protein
- 2.7g Fiber

Spicy and Peppery Fried Tofu

Preparation Time: 10 minutes

Cooking Time: 20 minutes

Serving: 2

Ingredients:

- 2 bell peppers, deveined and sliced
- 1 chili pepper, deveined and sliced
- 1 ½ tablespoons almond meal
- Salt and pepper, to taste
- 1 teaspoon ginger-garlic paste
- 1 teaspoon onion powder
- 6 ounces extra-firm tofu, pressed and cubed
- 1/2 teaspoon ground bay leaf
- 1 tablespoon sesame oil

Directions:

1. Toss your tofu, with almond meal, salt, pepper, ginger-garlic paste, onion powder, ground bay leaf.
2. In a sauté pan, heat the sesame oil over medium-high heat.
3. Fry the tofu cubes along with the peppers for about 6 minutes.

Nutrition:

- 223 Calories
- 15.9g Fat
- 15.6g Protein
- 3.3g Fiber

Colorful Creamy Soup

Preparation Time: 10 minutes

Cooking Time: 25 minutes

Serving: 6

Ingredients:

- 2 cups Swiss chard, torn into pieces
- Sea salt and pepper, to taste
- 2 thyme sprigs, chopped
- 2 teaspoons sesame oil
- 1 onion, chopped - 2 bay leaves
- 6 cups vegetable broth
- 1 cup grape tomatoes, chopped
- 1 cup almond milk, unflavored
- 1 teaspoon garlic, minced
- 2 celery stalks, chopped
- 1 zucchini, chopped
- 1/2 cup scallions, chopped

Directions:

1. In a heavy bottomed pot, heat the sesame oil in over a moderately-high heat. Sauté the onion, garlic, and celery, until they've softened. Add in the zucchini, Swiss chard, salt, pepper, thyme, bay leaves, broth,

and tomatoes; bring to a rapid boil. Turn the heat to a simmer.

2. Leave the lid slightly ajar and continue to simmer for about 13 minutes. Add in the almond milk and scallions; continue to cook for 4 minutes more or until thoroughly warmed.

Nutrition:

- 142 Calories
- 11.4g Fat
- 2.9g Protein
- 1.3g Fiber

Tofu Stuffed Zucchini

Preparation Time: 20 minutes

Cooking Time: 50 minutes Serving: 4

Ingredients:

- 4 zucchinis, cut into halves lengthwise and scoop out the pulp
- 6 ounces firm tofu, drained and crumbled
- 2 garlic cloves, pressed
- 1/2 cup onions, chopped
- 1 tablespoon olive oil
- 1 cup tomato puree
- 1 tablespoon nutritional yeast
- 2 ounces pecans, chopped
- 1/4 teaspoon curry powder
- Sea salt and pepper, to taste

Directions:

1. In a saucepan, heat the olive oil over a moderately-high heat; cook the tofu, garlic, and onion for about 5 minutes.
2. Stir in the tomato puree and scooped zucchini pulp; add all seasonings and continue to cook for a further 5 to 6 minutes.

3. Spoon the filling into the zucchini "shells" and arrange them in a lightly greased baking dish.
4. Bake in the preheated oven at 365 degrees F for 25 to 30 minutes. Top with nutritional yeast and pecans nuts; bake for a further 5 minutes.

Nutrition:

- 208 Calories
- 14.4g Fat
- 6.5g Protein
- 4.3g Fiber

Broccoli Masala

Preparation Time: 5 minutes

Cooking Time: 15 minutes

Serving: 4

Ingredients:

- 1/4 cup sesame oil
- 1-pound broccoli florets
- 1/2 teaspoon Garam Masala
- 1 tablespoon Kasuri Methi (dried fenugreek leaves)
- 1 Badi Elaichi (black cardamom)
- 1 teaspoon garlic, pressed
- Salt and pepper, to taste

Directions:

1. Parboil the broccoli for 6 to 7 minutes until it is crisp-tender.
2. Heat the sesame oil in a wok or saucepan until sizzling. Once hot, cook your broccoli for 3 to 4 minutes. Add in the other ingredients and give it a quick stir.
3. Adjust the spices to suit your taste.

Nutrition:

- 100 Calories
- 8.2g Fat
- 3.7g Protein
- 4g Fiber

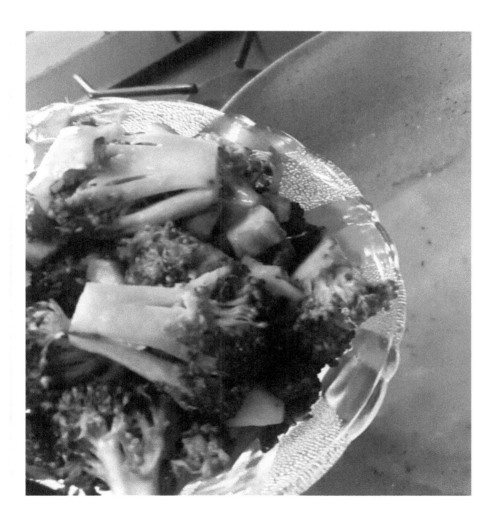

Italian-Style Tomato Crisps

Preparation Time: 10 minutes

Cooking Time: 5 hours

Serving: 6

Ingredients:

- 1 tablespoon Italian spice mix
- 1 ½ pounds Romano tomatoes, sliced
- 1/4 cup extra-virgin olive oil
- For Vegan Parmesan:
- 1/4 cup sunflower seeds
- Salt and pepper, to taste
- 1/4 teaspoon dried dill weed
- 1 teaspoon garlic powder
- 1/4 cup sesame seeds
- 1 tablespoon nutritional yeast

Directions:

1. Process all ingredients for the vegan parmesan in your food processor.
2. Toss the sliced tomatoes with the extra-virgin olive oil, Italian spice mix, and vegan parmesan.
3. Arrange the tomato slices on a parchment-lined baking sheet in a single layer. Bake at 220 degrees F about 5 hours.

Nutrition:

- 161 Calories
- 14g Fat
- 4.6g Protein
- 2.6g Fiber

Lebanese Asparagus with Baba Ghanoush

Preparation Time: 15 minutes

Cooking Time: 45 minutes

Serving: 6

Ingredients:

- 1/4 cup sesame oil
- 1 ½ pounds asparagus spears, med
- 1/2 teaspoon red pepper flakes
- Salt and pepper, to taste
- For Baba Ghanoush:
- 2 tablespoons fresh lime juice
- 2 teaspoons olive oil
- 1/2 cup onion, chopped
- 3/4-pound eggplant
- 1 teaspoon garlic, minced
- 1 tablespoon sesame paste
- 1/2 teaspoon allspice
- 1/4 teaspoon ground nutmeg
- 1/4 cup fresh parsley leaves, chopped
- Salt and ground black pepper, to taste

Directions:

1. Toss the asparagus spears with sesame oil, salt, and pepper. Arrange the asparagus spears on a foil-lined baking pan.

2. Roast in the preheated oven at 380 degrees F for 8 to 10 minutes.

3. Meanwhile, make your Baba Ghanoush. Bake eggplants in the preheated oven at 420 degrees F for 25 to 30 minutes; discard the skin and stems. In a saucepan, heat 2 the olive oil over a moderately-high heat. Cook the onion and garlic until tender and fragrant; heat off.

4. Add the roasted eggplant, sautéed onion mixture, sesame paste, lime juice, and spices to your blender or food processor. Pulse until creamy and smooth.

Nutrition:

- 149 Calories
- 12.1g Fat
- 3.6g Protein
- 4.6g Fiber

Garlic Mozzarella Bread

Preparation Time: 20 minutes

Cooking Time: 65 minutes

Serving: 8

Ingredients:

- 1 cup vegan mozzarella
- 1 cup almond flour
- ½ medium onion (diced)
- 4 tbsp. ground flaxseed
- 3 tbsp. olive oil
- ½ cup water
- 1 tbsp. Italian herbs
- ½ tsp. baking powder
- 2 garlic cloves (minced)
- Optional: ¼ cup black olives

Directions:

1. Preheat the oven to 350°F/175°C and line a large loaf pan with parchment paper. In a small bowl, combine the water with the ground flaxseed. Let the flaxseed soak for about 10 minutes.
2. Put the soaked seeds in a food processor with all the other ingredients, and pulse until they are combined into a smooth batter. Scrape the sides of the food

processor if necessary. Transfer the batter onto the loaf pan and let the mixture sit for a few minutes.

3. Put the loaf pan in the oven and bake the bread for 50 minutes, until the bread is firm and browned on top. Take the loaf pan out of the oven and allow the bread to cool down completely.

4. Transfer the bread to a cutting board and slice it into 8 slices. Serve and enjoy!

5. Alternatively, store the bread in an airtight container in the fridge and consume within 4 days. Store for a maximum of 60 days in the freezer and thaw at room temperature before serving.

Nutrition:

- 256 Calories
- 23.5 g. Fat
- 6.6 g. Protein

Truffle Parmesan Bread

Preparation Time: 20 minutes

Cooking Time: 65 minutes

Serving: 8

Ingredients:

- 1 cup truffle parmesan cheese
- 1 cup almond flour
- ½ cup button mushrooms (diced)
- 2 tbsp. soy sauce
- ½ medium onion (finely chopped)
- ½ cup ground flaxseed
- 4 tbsp. olive oil
- ½ cup water
- 1 tsp. dried thyme
- 1 tsp. dried basil
- 1 tsp. black pepper
- ½ tsp. baking powder

Directions:

1. Preheat the oven to 350°F/175°C and line a large loaf pan with parchment paper. In a small bowl, combine the water with the ground flaxseed. Let the flaxseed soak for about 10 minutes.

2. Meanwhile, put a medium-sized frying pan over medium-high heat and add a tablespoon of olive oil. When the oil is warm, add the chopped onions, mushrooms, and soy sauce to the frying pan and stir-fry until the mushrooms and onion have softened.

3. Put the flaxseed, stir-fried ingredients, and all remaining ingredients in a food processor and pulse until all ingredients are combined into a smooth mixture. Scrape down the sides of the food processor if necessary.

4. Transfer the mixture into the loaf pan and let the mixture sit for a few minutes. Put the loaf pan in the oven and bake the bread for about 50 minutes, until the bread is firm and browned on top.

5. Take the loaf pan out of the oven and allow the bread to cool down completely. Transfer the bread to a cutting board and slice it into 8 slices. Serve warm or cold and enjoy!

6. Alternatively, store the bread in an airtight container in the fridge and consume within 4 days.

7. Store for a maximum of 60 days in the freezer and thaw at room temperature before serving.

Nutrition:

- 296 Calories
- 26.9 g. Fat
- 7.7 g. Protein

Cauliflower Side Salad

Preparation Time: 14 minutes

Cooking Time: 7 minutes

Servings: 8

Ingredients:

- 21 oz. cauliflower
- 1 tbsp. water
- 4 boiled eggs, peeled and chopped
- 1 cup onion, chopped
- 1 cup celery, chopped
- 1 cup mayonnaise
- Salt and ground black pepper to taste
- 2 tbsp. cider vinegar
- 1 tsp. sucralose

Directions:

1. Divide cauliflower into florets and put them in heatproof bowl. Add water and place in microwave, cook for 5 minutes. Transfer to serving bowl.
2. Add eggs, onions, and celery. Stir gently.
3. In another bowl, whisk together mayonnaise, black pepper, salt, vinegar and sucralose. Add this sauce to salad and toss to coat. Serve.

Nutrition:

- 209 Calories
- 2.9g Carbs
- 19.7g Fat
- 3.97g Protein

Truffle Parmesan Salad

Preparation Time: 10 minutes

Cooking Time: 15 minutes

Serving: 4

Ingredients:

- 4 cups kale (chopped)
- ½ cup truffle parmesan cheese
- 1 tsp. Dijon mustard
- 2 tbsp. olive oil
- 2 tbsp. lemon juice
- Salt and pepper to taste
- Optional: 2 tbsp. water

Directions:

1. Rinse the kale with cold water, then drain the kale and put it into a large bowl. In a medium-sized bowl, mix the remaining ingredients into a dressing. Pour the dressing over the kale and stir gently to cover the kale evenly.
2. Transfer the large bowl to the fridge and allow the salad to chill for up to one hour – doing so will guarantee a better flavor. Alternatively, the salad can be served right away. Enjoy!

3. Alternatively, store the salad in the fridge using an airtight container and consume within 2 days.

Nutrition:

- 199 Calories
- 16.6 g Fat
- 3.5 g. Protein
- 1.9 g. Fiber

Cashew Siam Salad

Preparation Time: 10 minutes

Cooking Time: 15 minutes

Serving: 4

Ingredients:

Salad:

- 4 cups baby spinach (rinsed, drained)
- ½ cup pickled red cabbage

Dressing:

- 1-inch piece ginger (finely chopped)
- 1 tsp. chili garlic paste
- 1 tbsp. soy sauce
- ½ tbsp. rice vinegar
- 1 tbsp. sesame oil
- 3 tbsp. avocado oil
- Toppings:
- ½ cup raw cashews (unsalted)
- Optional: ¼ cup fresh cilantro (chopped)

Directions:

1. Put the spinach and red cabbage in a large bowl. Toss to combine and set the salad aside. Toast the cashews in a frying pan over medium-high heat, stirring

occasionally until the cashews are golden brown. This should take about 3 minutes. Turn off the heat and set the frying pan aside.

2. Mix all the dressing ingredients in medium-sized bowl and use a spoon to mix them into a smooth dressing. Pour the dressing over the spinach salad and top with the toasted cashews.

3. Toss the salad to combine all ingredients and transfer the large bowl to the fridge. Allow the salad to chill for up to one hour – doing so will guarantee a better flavor.

4. Alternatively, the salad can be served right away, topped with the optional cilantro. Enjoy!

5. Alternatively, store the salad in the fridge using an airtight container and consume within 2 days.

Nutrition:

- 236 Calories
- 21.6 g. Fat
- 4.2 g. Protein
- 1.3 g. Fiber

Avocado and Cauliflower Hummus

Preparation Time: 10 minutes

Cooking Time: 20 minutes

Serving: 2

Ingredients:

- 1 medium cauliflower (stem removed and chopped)
- 1 large Hass avocado (peeled, pitted, and chopped)
- ¼ cup extra virgin olive oil
- 2 garlic cloves
- ½ tbsp. lemon juice
- ½ tsp. onion powder
- Sea salt and ground black pepper to taste
- 2 large carrots (peeled and cut into fries, or use store-bought raw carrot fries)
- Optional: ¼ cup fresh cilantro (chopped)

Directions:

1. Preheat the oven to 450°F/220°C, and line a baking tray with aluminum foil. Put the chopped cauliflower on the baking tray and drizzle with 2 tablespoons of olive oil.
2. Roast the chopped cauliflower in the oven for 20-25 minutes, until lightly brown. Remove the tray from the oven and allow the cauliflower to cool down.

3. Add all the ingredients—except the carrots and optional fresh cilantro—to a food processor or blender, and blend the ingredients into a smooth hummus. Transfer the hummus to a medium-sized bowl, cover, and put it in the fridge for at least 30 minutes.

4. Take the hummus out of the fridge and, if desired, top it with the optional chopped cilantro and more salt and pepper to taste; serve with the carrot fries, and enjoy!

5. Alternatively, store it in the fridge in an airtight container, and consume within 2 days

Nutrition:

- 416 Calories
- 40.3g. Fat
- 3.3g. Protein
- 10.3g. Fiber

Italian Stuffed Mushrooms

Preparation Time: 10 minutes

Cooking Time: 35 minutes

Servings: 4

Ingredients:

- 1-pound button mushrooms, stems removed
- 2 tablespoons coconut oil, melted
- 1-pound broccoli florets
- 1 Italian pepper, chopped
- 1 teaspoon Italian herb mix
- Salt and pepper, to taste
- 1 shallot, finely chopped
- 2 garlic cloves, minced
- 1 cup vegan parmesan

Directions:

3. Parboil the broccoli in a large pot of salted water until crisp-tender, about 6 minutes. Mash the broccoli florets with a potato masher. In a saucepan, melt the coconut oil over a moderately-high heat. Once hot, cook the shallot, garlic, and pepper until tender and fragrant. Season with the spices and add in the broccoli.

4. Fill the mushroom cups with the broccoli mixture and bake in the preheated oven at 365 degrees F for about 10 minutes. Top with the vegan parmesan and bake for 10 minutes more or until it melts.

Nutrition:

- 206 Calories
- 13.4g Fat
- 12.7g Protein
- 4g Fiber

One-Pot Mushroom Stroganoff

Preparation Time: 10 minutes

Cooking Time: 25 minutes

Serving: 4

Ingredients:

- 2 tablespoons canola oil
- 1 parsnip, chopped
- 1 cup fresh brown mushrooms, sliced
- 1 cup onions, chopped
- 2 garlic cloves, pressed
- 1/2 cup celery rib, chopped
- 1 teaspoon Hungarian paprika
- 3 ½ cups roasted vegetable broth
- 1 cup tomato puree
- 1 tablespoon flaxseed meal
- 2 tablespoons sherry wine
- 1 rosemary sprig, chopped
- 1/2 teaspoon dried basil
- 1/2 teaspoon dried oregano

Directions:

5. In a heavy-bottomed pot, heat the oil over a moderately-high flame. Cook the onion and garlic for 2 minutes or until tender and aromatic.
6. Add in the celery, parsnip, and mushrooms, and continue to cook until they've softened; reserve.
7. Add in the sherry wine to deglaze the bottom of your pot. Add in the seasonings, vegetable broth, and tomato puree.
8. Continue to simmer, partially covered, for 15 to 18 minutes. Add in the flaxseed meal and stir until the sauce has thickened.

Nutrition:

- 114 Calories
- 7.3g Fat
- 2.1g Protein 3.1g Fiber

Avocado with Pine Nuts

Preparation Time: 5 minutes

Cooking Time: 10 minutes

Serving: 4

Ingredients:

- 2 avocados, pitted and halved
- 1 tablespoon coconut aminos
- 1/2 teaspoon garlic, minced
- 1 teaspoon fresh lime juice
- Salt and pepper, to taste
- 5 ounces pine nuts, ground
- 1 celery stalk, chopped

Directions:

3. Thoroughly combine the avocado pulp with the pine nuts, celery, garlic, fresh lime juice, and coconut aminos. Season with salt and pepper to taste.
4. Spoon the filling into the avocado halves.

Nutrition:

- 263 Calories
- 24.8g Fat
- 3.5g Protein
- 6.1g Fiber

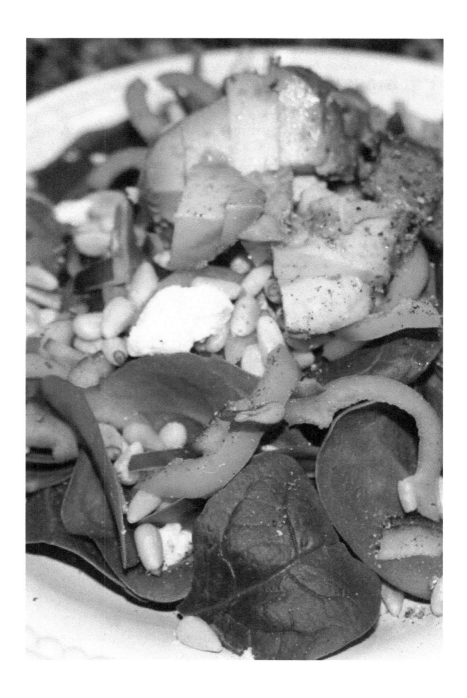

Zucchini Noodles with Famous Cashew Parmesan

Preparation Time: 5 minutes

Cooking Time: 15 minutes

Serving: 4

Ingredients:

For Zoodles:

- 2 tablespoons canola oil
- 4 zucchinis, peeled and sliced into noodle-shape strands
- Salt and pepper, to taste

For Cashew Parmesan:

- 1/2 cup raw cashews
- 1/4 teaspoon onion powder
- 1 garlic clove, minced
- 2 tablespoons nutritional yeast
- Sea salt and pepper, to taste

Directions:

4. In a saucepan, heat the canola oil over medium heat; once hot, cook your zoodles for 1 minute or so, stirring frequently to ensure even cooking.
5. Season with salt and pepper to taste.

6. In your food processor, process all ingredients for the cashew parmesan. Toss the cashew parmesan with the zoodles and enjoy!

Nutrition:

- 145 Calories
- 10.6g Fat
- 5.5g Protein
- 1.6g Fiber

Cream of Broccoli Soup

Preparation Time: 5 minutes

Cooking Time: 15 minutes

Serving: 4

Ingredients:

- 1-pound broccoli, cut into small florets
- 8 ounces baby spinach
- 4 cups roasted vegetable broth
- 2 tablespoons olive oil
- 1 yellow onion, chopped
- 2 garlic cloves, minced
- 1/2 cup coconut milk
- Salt and pepper, to taste
- 2 tablespoons parsley, chopped

Directions:

5. Heat the oil in a soup pot over a moderately-high flame. Then, sauté the onion and garlic until they're tender and fragrant.
6. Add in the broccoli, spinach, and broth; bring to a rolling boil. Immediately turn the heat to a simmer.
7. Pour in the coconut milk, salt, pepper, and parsley; continue to simmer, partially covered, until cooked through.

8. Puree your soup with an immersion blender.

Nutrition:

- 252 Calories20.3g Fat
- 8.1g Protein
- 4.5g Fiber

Swiss Chard Chips with Avocado Dip

Preparation Time: 10 minutes

Cooking Time: 20 minutes

Serving: 6

Ingredients:

- 1 tablespoon coconut oil
- Sea salt and pepper, to taste
- 2 cups Swiss chard, cleaned

Avocado Dip:

- 3 ripe avocados, pitted and mashed
- 2 garlic cloves, finely minced
- 2 tablespoons extra-virgin olive oil
- 2 teaspoons lemon juice
- Salt and pepper, to taste

Directions:

3. Toss the Swiss chard with the coconut oil, salt, and pepper. Bake the Swiss chard leaves in the preheated oven at 310 degrees F for about 10 minutes until the edges brown but are not burnt.
4. Thoroughly combine the ingredients for the avocado dip.

Nutrition:

- 269 Calories
- 26.7g Fat
- 2.3g Protein
- 4.1g Fiber

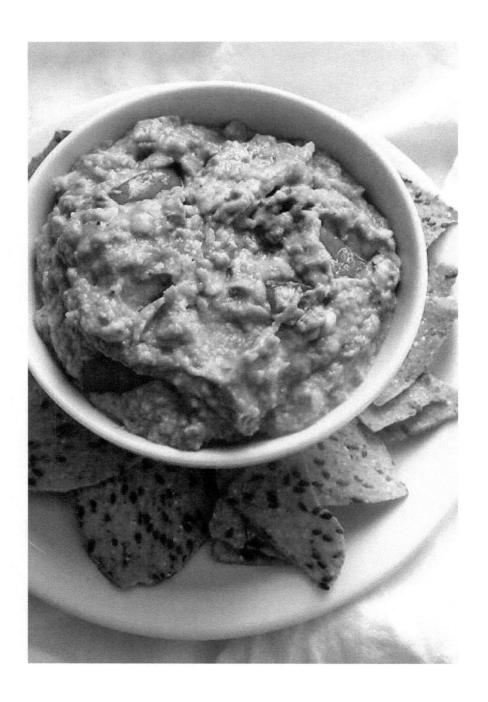

Banana Blueberry Smoothie

Preparation Time: 5 minutes

Cooking Time: 0 minutes

Serving: 4

Ingredients:

- 1/2 cup fresh blueberries
- 1/2 banana, peeled and sliced
- 1/2 cup water
- 1 ½ cups coconut milk
- 1 tablespoon vegan protein powder, zero carbs

Directions:

2. Blend all ingredients until creamy and uniform.

Nutrition:

- 247 Calories
- 21.7g Fat
- 2.6g Protein
- 3g Fiber

Cajun Artichoke with Tofu

Preparation Time: 15 minutes

Cooking Time: 30 minutes

Serving: 4

Ingredients:

- 1-pound artichokes, trimmed and cut into pieces
- 2 tablespoons coconut oil, room temperature
- 1 block tofu, pressed and cubed
- 1 teaspoon fresh garlic, minced
- 1 teaspoon Cajun spice mix
- 1 Spanish pepper, chopped
- 1/4 cup vegetable broth
- Salt and pepper, to taste

Directions:

4. Parboil your artichokes in a pot of lightly salted water for 13 to 15 minutes or until they're crisp-tender; drain.

5. In a large saucepan, melt the coconut oil over medium-high heat; fry the tofu cubes for 5 to 6 minutes or until golden-brown.

6. Add in the garlic, Cajun spice mix, Spanish pepper, broth, salt, and pepper. Add in the reserved artichokes and continue to cook until for 5 minutes more.

Nutrition:

- 138 Calories
- 8.9g Fat
- 6.4g Protein
- 5g Fiber

Mushroom and Cauliflower Medley

Preparation Time: 15 minutes

Cooking Time: 30 minutes

Serving: 4

Ingredients:

- 8 ounces brown mushrooms, halved
- 1 head cauliflower, cut into florets
- 1/4 cup olive oil
- 1/2 teaspoon turmeric powder
- 1 teaspoon garlic, smashed
- 1 cup tomato, pureed
- Salt and pepper, to taste

Directions:

3. Toss all ingredients in a lightly oiled baking pan.
4. Roast the vegetable in the preheated oven at 380 degrees F for 25 to 30 minutes.

Nutrition:

- 113 Calories
- 6.7g Fat
- 5g Protein
- 2.7g Fiber

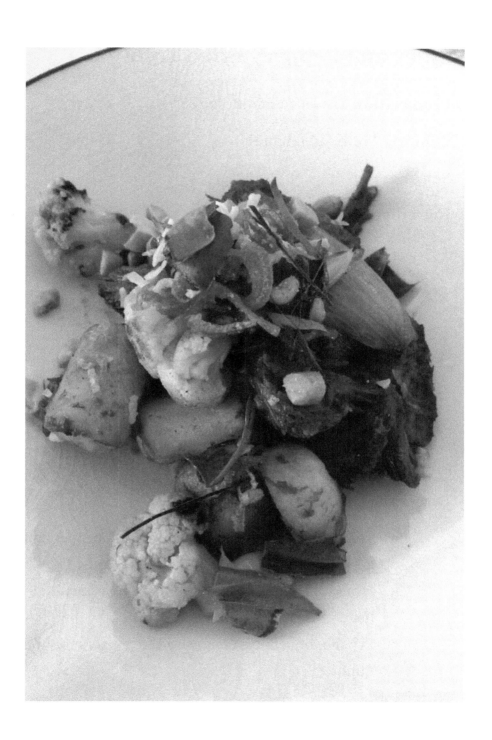

Spicy and Peppery Fried Tofu

Preparation Time: 10 minutes

Cooking Time: 20 minutes

Serving: 2

Ingredients:

- 2 bell peppers, deveined and sliced
- 1 chili pepper, deveined and sliced
- 1 ½ tablespoons almond meal
- Salt and pepper, to taste
- 1 teaspoon ginger-garlic paste
- 1 teaspoon onion powder
- 6 ounces extra-firm tofu, pressed and cubed
- 1/2 teaspoon ground bay leaf
- 1 tablespoon sesame oil

Directions:

4. Toss your tofu, with almond meal, salt, pepper, ginger-garlic paste, onion powder, ground bay leaf.
5. In a sauté pan, heat the sesame oil over medium-high heat.
6. Fry the tofu cubes along with the peppers for about 6 minutes.

Nutrition:

- 223 Calories
- 15.9g Fat
- 15.6g Protein
- 3.3g Fiber

Colorful Creamy Soup

Preparation Time: 10 minutes

Cooking Time: 25 minutes

Serving: 6

Ingredients:

- 2 cups Swiss chard, torn into pieces
- Sea salt and pepper, to taste
- 2 thyme sprigs, chopped
- 2 teaspoons sesame oil
- 1 onion, chopped - 2 bay leaves
- 6 cups vegetable broth
- 1 cup grape tomatoes, chopped
- 1 cup almond milk, unflavored
- 1 teaspoon garlic, minced
- 2 celery stalks, chopped
- 1 zucchini, chopped
- 1/2 cup scallions, chopped

Directions:

3. In a heavy bottomed pot, heat the sesame oil in over a moderately-high heat. Sauté the onion, garlic, and celery, until they've softened. Add in the zucchini, Swiss chard, salt, pepper, thyme, bay leaves, broth,

and tomatoes; bring to a rapid boil. Turn the heat to a simmer.

4. Leave the lid slightly ajar and continue to simmer for about 13 minutes. Add in the almond milk and scallions; continue to cook for 4 minutes more or until thoroughly warmed.

Nutrition:

- 142 Calories
- 11.4g Fat
- 2.9g Protein
- 1.3g Fiber

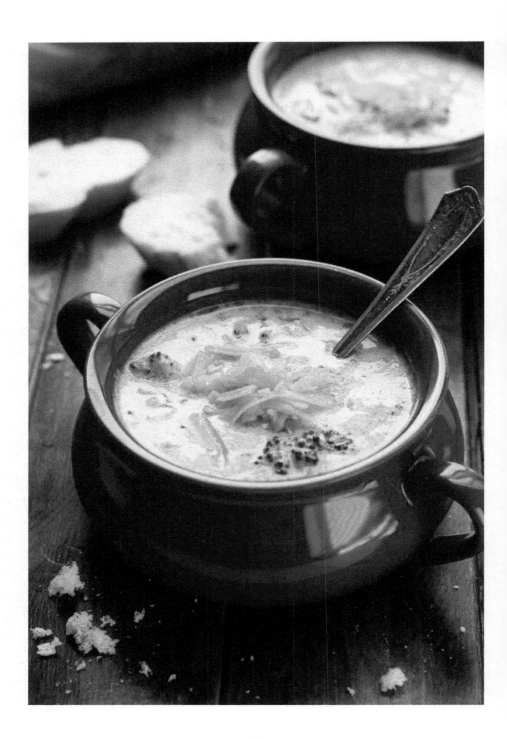

Lunch Caesar Salad

Preparation Time: 15 minutes

Cooking time: 10 minutes

Servings: 2

Ingredients:

- 1 avocado, pitted
- 1 chicken breast, grilled and shredded
- 1 cup bacon, cooked and crumbled
- 3 tbsp. creamy Caesar dressing
- Salt and ground black pepper to taste

Directions:

1. Peel and slice avocado. In medium bowl, combine bacon, chicken breast and avocado.
2. Add creamy Cesar dressing, stir well. Season with salt and pepper, stir. Serve.

Nutrition:

- 329 Calories
- 2.99g Carbs
- 22.9g Fat
- 17.8g Protein

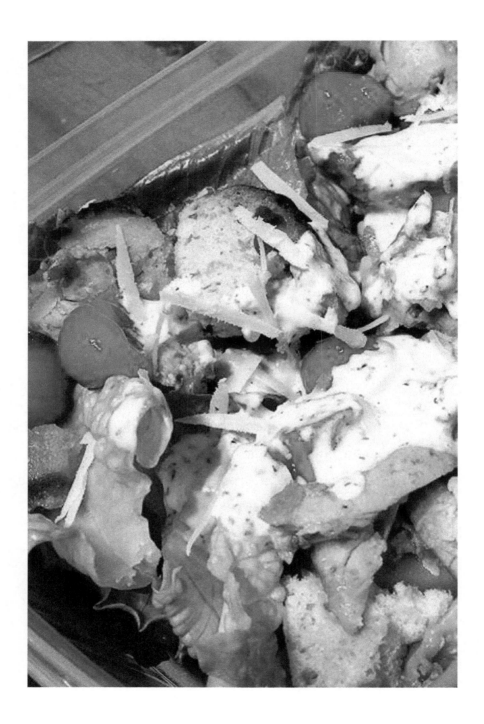

Asian Side Salad

Preparation Time: 35 minutes

Cooking Time: 12 minutes

Servings: 4

Ingredients:

- 1 green onion
- 1 cucumber
- 2 tbsp. coconut oil
- 1 packet Asian noodles, cooked
- ¼ tsp. red pepper flakes
- 1 tbsp. sesame oil
- 1 tbsp. balsamic vinegar
- 1 tsp. sesame seeds
- Salt and ground black pepper to taste

Directions:

1. Chop onion. Slice cucumber thin. Preheat pan with oil on medium high heat. Add cooked noodles and close lid.
2. Fry noodles for 5 minutes until crispy. Transfer noodles to paper towels and drain grease.
3. Combine cucumber, pepper flakes, green onion, sesame oil, vinegar, sesame seeds, pepper, salt and

noodles. Mix well. Put in refrigerator at least for 20-30 minutes. Serve.

Nutrition:

- 397 Calories 3.97g Carbs
- 33.7g Fat
- 1.98g Protein

Keto Egg Salad

Preparation Time: 15 minutes

Cooking Time: 10 minutes

Servings: 4

Ingredients:

- 6 oz. ham, chopped
- 5 eggs, boiled and chopped
- 1 tsp. garlic, minced
- ½ tsp. basil
- 1 tsp. oregano
- 1 tbsp. apple cider vinegar
- 1 tsp. kosher salt
- ½ cup cream cheese

Directions:

1. In medium bowl, combine chopped ham with chopped eggs, stir. In another bowl, mix together garlic, basil, oregano, vinegar, and salt. Stir the mixture till you get homogeneous consistency.
2. Whisk together spice mixture and cream cheese. Add cream cheese sauce to egg mixture and stir gently. Serve.

Nutrition:

- 341 Calories
- 26g Fat
- 22.1g Protein

Cobb Salad

Preparation Time: 20 minutes

Cooking Time: 27 minutes

Servings: 1

Ingredients:

- 1 tbsp. olive oil
- 4 oz. chicken breast
- 2 strips bacon
- 1 cup spinach, chopped roughly
- 1 large hard-boiled egg, peeled and chopped
- ¼ avocado, peeled and chopped
- ½ tsp. white vinegar

Directions:

1. Heat up pan on medium heat and add oil. Add chicken breast and bacon, cook until get desired crispiness.
2. Add spinach and egg, stir. Add avocado and mix well. Sprinkle with white vinegar and stir.
3. Serve.

Nutrition:

- 589Calories
- 47.8g Fat
- 42g Protein

Bacon and Zucchini Noodles Salad

Preparation Time: 15 minutes

Cooking Time: 10 minutes

Servings: 3

Ingredients:

- 32 oz. zucchini noodles
- 1 cup baby spinach
- 1/3 cup blue cheese, crumbled
- ½ cup bacon, cooked and crumbled
- 1/3 cup blue cheese dressing
- Ground black pepper to taste

Directions:

1. Combine zucchini noodles, spinach, blue cheese, and bacon, stir carefully.
2. Add black pepper and cheese dressing, toss to coat. Serve.

Nutrition:

- 198 Calories
- 13.9g Fat
- 9.95g Protein

Chicken Salad

Preparation Time: 15 minutes

Cooking Time: 10 minutes

Servings: 3

Ingredients:

- 1 celery stalk
- 2 tbsp. fresh parsley
- 1 green onion
- 5 oz. chicken breast, roasted and chopped
- 1 egg, hard-boiled, peeled and chopped
- Salt and ground black pepper to taste
- ½ tsp. garlic powder
- 1/3 cup mayonnaise
- 1 tsp. mustard
- ½ tbsp. dill relish

Directions:

1. Wash and chop celery, parsley and onion. Place celery, onion and parsley in blender or food processor and blend well. Remove this mass from food processor and set aside.

2. Place chicken in food processor and pulse well. Add chicken to onion mixture and stir. Add egg, pepper

and salt, stir gently. Add garlic powder, mayonnaise, and mustard and dill relish, toss to coat.

3. Serve.

Nutrition:

- 279 Calories
- 22.9g Fat
- 11.9g Protein

Asparagus Salad

Preparation Time: 20 minutes

Cooking Time: 5 minutes

Servings: 5

Ingredients:

- 2 lbs. asparagus, cooked and halved
- 1 tbsp. butter, melted
- ½ tsp. garlic powder
- 1 tsp. sesame seeds
- 1 tbsp. coconut oil
- 1 tbsp. apple cider vinegar
- 1 tsp. dried basil
- 1 tsp. salt
- 4 oz. Parmesan cheese, grated

Directions:

1. In bowl, combine asparagus, butter and garlic powder. Stir well. Add sesame seeds, coconut oil, vinegar, basil and salt. Mix well.
2. Set salad aside to marinate. Serve salad with grated Parmesan cheese.

Nutrition:

- 133 Calories

- 8.85g Fat
- 10g Protein

Apple Salad

Preparation Time: 15 minutes

Cooking Time: 5 minutes

Servings: 4

Ingredients:

- 1 medium apple
- 2 oz. pecans
- 16 oz. broccoli florets
- 1 green onion
- 2 tsp. poppy seeds
- Salt and ground black pepper to taste
- ¼ cup sour cream
- ¼ cup mayonnaise
- ½ tsp. lemon juice
- 1 tsp. apple cider vinegar

Directions:

1. Core and grate apple. Chop pecans and broccoli florets. Dice green onion. In bowl, combine broccoli, apple, pecans, and green onion. Stir well.
2. Sprinkle with poppy seeds, black pepper and salt, stir carefully. In another bowl, whisk sour cream, mayonnaise, lemon juice and vinegar.
3. Add this mixture to salad and toss to coat. Serve.

Nutrition:

- 249 Calories
- 22.9g Fat
- 4.8g Protein

Bok Choy Salad

Preparation Time: 20 minutes

Cooking Time: 10 minutes

Servings: 6

Ingredients:

- 10 oz. bok choy, chopped roughly
- 2 tbsp. coconut oil
- 4 tbsp. chicken stock
- 1 tsp. basil
- 1 tsp. ground black pepper
- 1 white onion, peeled and sliced
- ¼ cup white mushrooms, marinated and chopped
- 1 lb. tofu, chopped
- 1 tsp. oregano
- 1 tsp. almond milk

Directions:

1. Heat up pan on medium heat. Add bok choy, 1 tablespoon of oil and chicken stock.
2. Season with basil and black pepper. Add onion and close lid.
3. Simmer vegetables for 5-6 minutes, stirring constantly. Transfer vegetables to bowl and add

mushrooms. Pour 1 tablespoon of oil in pan and heat it up again.

4. Add chopped tofu and cook for 2 minutes. Transfer tofu to bowl with vegetables and sprinkle with oregano. Pour in almond milk and toss to coat.

5. Serve salad.

Nutrition:

- 130 Calories
- 4.67g Carbs
- 11g Fat
- 6.9g Protein

Halloumi Salad

Preparation Time: 15 minutes

Cooking Time: 12 minutes

Servings: 2

Ingredients:

- 3 oz. halloumi cheese, sliced
- 1 cucumber, sliced
- ½ cup baby arugula
- 5 cherry tomatoes, halved
- 1 oz. walnuts, chopped
- Salt and ground black pepper to taste
- ½ tsp. olive oil
- ¼ tsp. balsamic vinegar

Directions:

1. Preheat grill on medium high heat. Put halloumi cheese in grill and cook for 5 minutes per side.
2. In mixing bowl, combine cucumber, arugula, tomatoes, and walnuts. Place halloumi pieces on top.
3. Sprinkle with black pepper and salt. Drizzle oil and balsamic vinegar, toss to coat.
4. Serve.

Nutrition:

- 448 Calories
- 3.98g Carbs
- 42.8g Fat
- 22.3g Protein

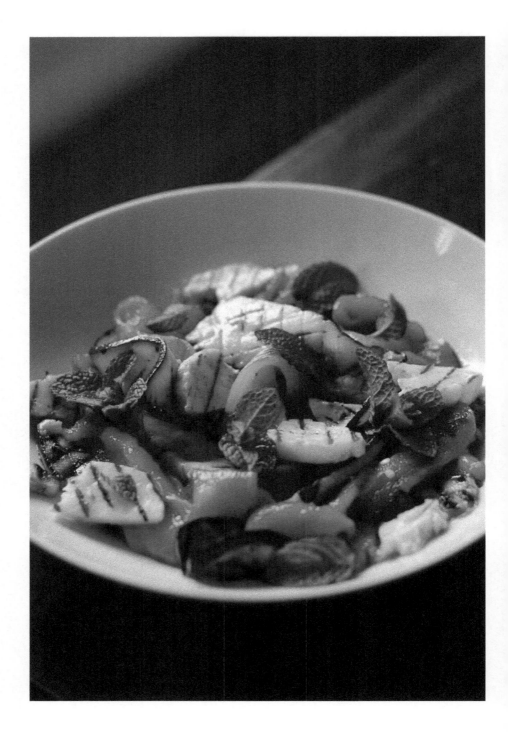

Smoked Salmon Salad

Preparation Time: 17 minutes

Cooking Time: 10 minutes

Servings: 4

Ingredients:

- 8 oz. smoked salmon, sliced into thin pieces
- 2 oz. pecans, crushed
- 3 medium tomatoes, chopped
- ½ cup lettuce, chopped
- 1 cucumber, diced
- 1/3 cup cream cheese
- 1/3 cup coconut milk
- ½ tsp. oregano
- 1 tbsp. lemon juice, chopped
- ½ tsp. basil
- 1 tsp. salt

Directions:

1. In medium bowl, combine salmon with pecans and stir. Add tomatoes, lettuce and cucumber, stir well.
2. In another bowl, mix together cream cheese, coconut milk, oregano, lemon juice, basil and salt. Stir mixture until get homogenous mass. Serve salmon salad with cream cheese sauce.

Nutrition:

- 211 Calories
- 15.9g Fat
- 9.95g Protein

Keto Tricolor Salad

Preparation Time: 12 minutes

Cooking Time: 8 minutes

Servings: 5

Ingredients:

- 5 oz. mozzarella cheese
- 1 tsp. oregano
- 1 tsp. minced garlic
- 1 tsp. basil
- 1 tbsp. coconut oil
- 1 tsp. lemon juice
- 2 medium tomatoes, sliced
- 7 oz. avocado, pitted and sliced
- 8 olives, pitted and sliced

Directions:

1. Cut mozzarella cheese balls into halves. In medium bowl, mix together oregano, garlic, basil, coconut oil and lemon juice.
2. On serving plate place sliced tomato, then place sliced avocado and olives. Put mozzarella pieces on top. Drizzle coconut sauce over salad and serve.

Nutrition:

- 239 Calories
- 7.9g Carbs
- 20.1g Fat
- 11.77g Protein

Caprese Salad

Preparation Time: 7 minutes

Cooking Time: 10 minutes

Servings: 2

Ingredients:

- 8 oz. mozzarella cheese
- 1 medium tomato
- 4 basil leaves
- Salt and ground black pepper to taste
- 3 tsp. balsamic vinegar
- 1 tbsp. olive oil

Directions:

1. Slice mozzarella cheese and tomato. Torn basil leaves. Alternate tomato and mozzarella slices on 2 plates. Season with pepper and salt. Drizzle vinegar and olive oil. Sprinkle with the basil leaves.
2. Serve.

Nutrition:

- 148 Calories
- 5.9g Carbs
- 11.8g Fat
- 8.95g Protein

Warm Bacon Salad

Preparation Time: 16 minutes

Cooking Time: 18 minutes

Servings: 5

Ingredients:

- 16 oz. bacon strips, chopped
- 1 tsp. cilantro
- 1 tsp. ground ginger
- 1 tsp. kosher salt
- 2 tbsp. butter
- 3 boiled eggs, peeled and chopped
- 2 tomatoes, diced
- 1 oz. spinach, chopped
- 4 oz. Cheddar cheese, grated
- 1 tsp. almond milk
- 7 oz. eggplant, peeled and diced

Directions:

1. In medium bowl, combine bacon, cilantro, ginger and salt. Heat up pan over medium heat and melt 1 tablespoon of butter.
2. Put bacon in pan and cook for 5 minutes. Transfer bacon to plate.

3. Meanwhile, in bowl, mix together chopped eggs, tomatoes and spinach. Sprinkle with cheese and add almond milk. Heat up pan again over medium heat and melt remaining 1 tablespoon of butter.

4. Add diced eggplants and fry for 8 minutes, stirring occasionally. Then add bacon and roasted eggplants to salad. Season with salt and stir gently. Serve.

Nutrition:

- 159 Calories
- 4.22g Carbs
- 13g Fat
- 8.75g Protein

Cauliflower Side Salad

Preparation Time: 14 minutes

Cooking Time: 7 minutes

Servings: 8

Ingredients:

- 21 oz. cauliflower
- 1 tbsp. water
- 4 boiled eggs, peeled and chopped
- 1 cup onion, chopped
- 1 cup celery, chopped
- 1 cup mayonnaise
- Salt and ground black pepper to taste
- 2 tbsp. cider vinegar
- 1 tsp. sucralose

Directions:

3. Divide cauliflower into florets and put them in heatproof bowl. Add water and place in microwave, cook for 5 minutes. Transfer to serving bowl.
4. Add eggs, onions, and celery. Stir gently.
4. In another bowl, whisk together mayonnaise, black pepper, salt, vinegar and sucralose. Add this sauce to salad and toss to coat. Serve.

Nutrition:

- 209 Calories
- 2.9g Carbs
- 19.7g Fat
- 3.97g Protein

Keto Tricolor Salad

Preparation Time: 12 minutes

Cooking Time: 8 minutes

Servings: 5

Ingredients:

- 5 oz. mozzarella cheese
- 1 tsp. oregano
- 1 tsp. minced garlic
- 1 tsp. basil
- 1 tbsp. coconut oil
- 1 tsp. lemon juice
- 2 medium tomatoes, sliced
- 7 oz. avocado, pitted and sliced
- 8 olives, pitted and sliced

Directions:

3. Cut mozzarella cheese balls into halves. In medium bowl, mix together oregano, garlic, basil, coconut oil and lemon juice.
4. On serving plate place sliced tomato, then place sliced avocado and olives. Put mozzarella pieces on top. Drizzle coconut sauce over salad and serve.

Nutrition:

- 239 Calories
- 7.9g Carbs
- 20.1g Fat
- 11.77g Protein

Low Carb Chicken Salad with Chimichurri Sauce

Preparation Time: 10 minutes

Cooking Time: 15 minutes

Serving: 5

Ingredients:

- 250 grams of various lettuce leaves
- 2 medium chicken breasts
- 2 medium avocados
- ¼ cup olive oil
- 3 tablespoons red wine vinegar
- ¼ cup parsley
- 1 tablespoon oregano
- 1 teaspoon chili pepper
- 1 teaspoon garlic

Directions:

1. Preheat the non-stick skillet. Place the lettuce and diced avocado in a salad bowl. Cook the chicken breasts, fry them until white. Let the chicken cool.
2. In a small bowl, combine olive oil, vinegar, parsley, oregano, garlic, and chili. Cut the chicken breast into

cubes. Add the chopped chicken fillet to the salad and season with the classic chimichurri sauce.

3. Garnish the salad with additional chimichurri sauce and serve.

Nutrition:

- 285.94 calories
- 21.24 g fat
- 17.24 g protein.

Potluck Lamb Salad

Preparation Time: 20 minutes

Cooking Time: 10 minutes

Servings: 4

Ingredients:

- 2 tbsp. olive oil, divided
- 12 oz. grass-fed lamb leg steaks
- 6½ oz. halloumi cheese
- 2 jarred roasted red bell peppers
- 2 cucumbers, cut into thin ribbons
- 3 C. fresh baby spinach
- 2 tbsp. balsamic vinegar

Directions:

1. In a skillet, heat 1 tbsp. of the oil over medium-high heat and cook the lamb steaks for about 4-5 minutes per side or until desired doneness. Transfer the lamb steaks onto a cutting board for about 5 minutes. Then cut the lamb steaks into thin slices. In the same skillet, add haloumi and cook for about 1-2 minutes per side or until golden.

2. In a salad bowl, add the lamb, haloumi, bell pepper, cucumber, salad leaves, vinegar, and remaining oil and toss to combine.

3. Serve immediately.

Nutrition:

- 420 Calories
- 35.4g Protein
- 1.3g Fiber

Spring Supper Salad

Preparation Time: 15 minutes

Cooking Time: 5 minutes

Servings: 5

Ingredients:

For Salad:

- 1 lb. fresh asparagus
- ½ lb. smoked salmon
- 2 heads red leaf lettuce
- ¼ C. pecans

For Dressing:

- ¼ C. olive oil
- 2 tbsp. fresh lemon juice
- 1 tsp. Dijon mustard

Directions:

1. In a pan of boiling water, add the asparagus and cook for about 5 minutes. Drain the asparagus well. In a serving bowl, add the asparagus and remaining salad ingredients and mix. In another bowl, add all the dressing ingredients and beat until well combined. Place the dressing over salad and gently, toss to coat well. Serve immediately.

Nutrition:

- 223 Calories
- 8.5g Carbohydrates
- 3.5g Fiber

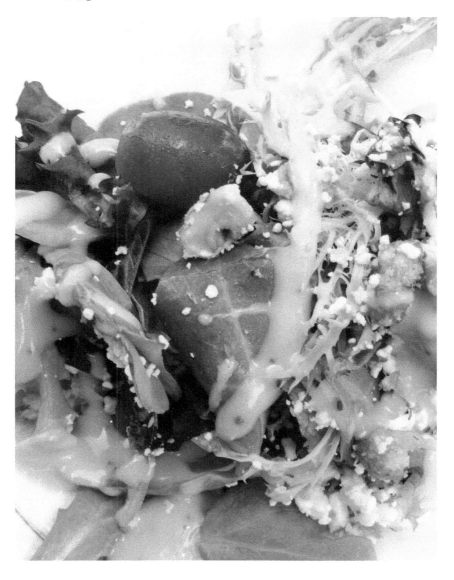

Chicken-of-Sea Salad

Preparation Time: 15 minutes

Cooking Time: 5 minutes

Servings: 6

Ingredients:

- 2 (6-oz.) cans olive oil-packed tuna
- 2 (6-oz.) cans water packed tuna
- ¾ C. mayonnaise
- 2 celery stalks
- ¼ of onion
- 1 tbsp. fresh lime juice
- 2 tbsp. mustard
- 6 C. fresh baby arugula

Directions:

1. In a large bowl, add all the ingredients except arugula and gently stir to combine. Divide arugula onto serving plates and top with tuna mixture. Serve immediately.

Nutrition:

- 325 Calories
- 27.4g Protein
- 1.1g Fiber

Lightning Source UK Ltd.
Milton Keynes UK
UKHW021013240621
386072UK00001B/88